C.H.E.M.O. Plan Your Day

C.H.E.M.O. Plan Your Day

Mamie L. Arms

iUniverse, Inc.
Bloomington

C.H.E.M.O. Plan Your Day

iUniverse books may be ordered through booksellers or by contacting:

iUniverse
1663 Liberty Drive
Bloomington, IN 47403
www.iuniverse.com
1-800-Authors (1-800-288-4677)

Because of the dynamic nature of the Internet, any web addresses or links contained in this book may have changed since publication and may no longer be valid. The views expressed in this work are solely those of the author and do not necessarily reflect the views of the publisher, and the publisher hereby disclaims any responsibility for them.

Any people depicted in stock imagery provided by Thinkstock are models, and such images are being used for illustrative purposes only.
Certain stock imagery © Thinkstock.

ISBN: 978-1-4620-2215-1 (sc)
ISBN: 978-1-4620-2216-8 (ebk)

Printed in the United States of America

iUniverse rev. date: 05/12/2011

To those who find they are faced with the treatment of Chemo.

TABLE OF CONTENTS

Foreword

You know with calendars it's so easy to look back over the year. I look over my yearly calendar and have noticed that I average five days out of the whole month that have no ink on those days. All other days have so much ink that I almost can't see the number in the block.

What does that tell me? I'm a busy person. I have always been a busy person. I love utilizing my time constructively accomplishing a ton of things. I need to be organized, know what I'm doing, where I'm going, who I'll meet or deal with for the day. Needing to know how I'll get there and get the job accomplished is for my satisfaction. I always have to feel that I have options (not what if's).

I have to always "plan my day". Let me emphasize planning the day. Well little did I know that I'd be planning so many days for one event in my life. I live to live a stress free life, which makes my story somewhat funny.

I'm trying to juggle three different doctors at a time figuring once I get one area fixed then the next area will follow suit. Hoping one appointment doesn't interfere with the other. Well they all eventually got fixed. Of the three, one was a very serious matter. I kept it on a small scale. I guess I still do.

September 2005, I was diagnosed with breast cancer. When the doctor told me I just said "Ok, what do we do now?" I had had this terrific doctor just a year before, with a benign mass which he removed. The year before that, I had encountered my first breast mass (benign also) removal.

So I'm in the middle of trying to reach my sixth month employment mark to enroll in the insurance plan at work that was a week later. I couldn't due to my "pre-existing" condition. I laughed. My luck.

Also at this time, I'm on pins and needles waiting for my first grandbaby. My daughter informs me it's a boy by way of the ultrasound. Ok so now I'm working, scheduling surgery, buying; planning on a grandson. I'm constantly checking my calendar.

Oh—let's throw in menopause while we're at it. Four days later I get the call. The baby is a girl! I hadn't laughed so hard in such a long time. I was so happy; nothing could ever take that joy away.

I get scheduled for my left breast mastectomy on Columbus Day (guess Columbus wasn't the only one to discover!). I worked all the way up to my surgery. I figured I might as well, I had to fast anyway. I planned that out. One night stay in the hospital then two weeks out of work, that's what the doctor told me. I received a lot of information to read and to answer any questions. I had noticed that a lot of info was left out of booklets and doctors offices.

I had learned to adjust a few things, as my Chemo went on. I will share with you the things I adjusted to and learned with a lot of humor. You have to laugh and realize "I refuse to let Chemo (cancer) run me. I'm in control".

This is "my day" not Chemo's (cancer). Let's get ready for your new journey through Chemo as you plan your day.

Things to Get You Started

Bedside table—Wal-Mart $20
Plunger or drain cleaner (For when your hair falls out.)
Get bills in order (How will you financially live for two—twelve months depending on you and length of your chemo.)
Pillows (To make you comfortable)
Puke bucket (To get sick in with a little water in it)
Remotes to electronics
Blender
Lots of liquids (Especially water)
Joyful/Inspiring pictures

Many of these items again are your choice such as the plunger or drain cleaner. You were told your hair more than likely will fall out, but did you think of the drains? I decided to just shave my head, due to the fact I didn't want a clogged drain. Not to mention my hair follicles hurt. One benefit to hair loss no shaving or hot wax. Out go the nose hairs, armpit hairs, etc. The blender has become my best friend next to prune juice. Pureed food meant no sore mouth.

First Aid Kit for Chemo

Tylenol
Band-Aids
Anti-diarrhea
Fiber Laxative
Eye Lubricant Drops
Eucerin Body Creme
Thera-Flu Cough and Cold
Prune Juice
Electric Shaver—hair hurts falling out

Private Thoughts

Private Thoughts

Private Thoughts

Private Thoughts

<u>Private Thoughts</u>

Private Thoughts

Express Yourself

Feel free to scribble and let out your emotions.

Express Yourself

Feel free to scribble and let out your emotions.

Express Yourself

Feel free to scribble and let out your emotions.

Express Yourself

Feel free to scribble and let out your emotions.

Express Yourself

Feel free to scribble and let out your emotions.

Important Phone Numbers

People that can run errands real quick for you.

_____ _____

_____ _____

_____ _____

_____ _____

_____ _____

_____ _____

_____ _____

_____ _____

_____ _____

Pharmacy: _____
Do they deliver?

Transportation

Public:

Senior Service:

Government Transportation:

Friend:

Grocery List

<u>Grocery List</u>

<u>Grocery List</u>

Grocery List

Grocery List

Medical Expenses

To Whom Paid   **Amount**

_____ _____

_____ _____

_____ _____

_____ _____

_____ _____

_____ _____

_____ _____

_____ _____

_____ _____

_____ _____

_____ _____

Medical Expenses

To Whom Paid	Amount
_____	_____
_____	_____
_____	_____
_____	_____
_____	_____
_____	_____
_____	_____
_____	_____
_____	_____
_____	_____
_____	_____
_____	_____

Medical Expenses

To Whom Paid   Amount

_____   _____

_____   _____

_____   _____

_____   _____

_____   _____

_____   _____

_____   _____

_____   _____

_____   _____

_____   _____

_____   _____

Medical Expenses

To WhomPaid   **Amount**

_____   _____

_____   _____

_____   _____

_____   _____

_____   _____

_____   _____

_____   _____

_____   _____

_____   _____

_____   _____

_____   _____

Medical Expenses

To Whom Paid   **Amount**

_____ _____

_____ _____

_____ _____

_____ _____

_____ _____

_____ _____

_____ _____

_____ _____

_____ _____

_____ _____

_____ _____

Medical Expenses

To Whom Paid	Amount
_____	_____
_____	_____
_____	_____
_____	_____
_____	_____
_____	_____
_____	_____
_____	_____
_____	_____
_____	_____
_____	_____

Medical Expenses

To Whom Paid	Amount
_____	_____
_____	_____
_____	_____
_____	_____
_____	_____
_____	_____
_____	_____
_____	_____
_____	_____
_____	_____
_____	_____

Medicines And Prescriptions

To Whom Paid   **Amount**

_____   _____

_____   _____

_____   _____

_____   _____

_____   _____

_____   _____

_____   _____

_____   _____

_____   _____

_____   _____

_____   _____

_____   _____

Medicines And Prescriptions

To Whom Paid   **Amount**

_____   _____

_____   _____

_____   _____

_____   _____

_____   _____

_____   _____

_____   _____

_____   _____

_____   _____

_____   _____

Things to Do When I'm Up

1. Food Shop
   - Freeze portioned foods so all you have to do is reheat.
   - Have handy snacks, according to your diet.
   - Your sense of taste may change along the way. A suggestion, keep an eye on expiration dates, and if you choose to puree your food keep in mind that your portions will be larger than if not. I also use broths for flavor and consistency. My first puree food was barbeque chicken (yum) with mash potatoes and jell-o for dessert.
2. Special Occasion Items
   - Sometimes I would make my own items which helped me feel relaxed and keep my mind off treatment.
3. Picture Taking
   - You seem to see things in a different light. I took a picture of myself when I was bald. (I was looking good!!)
4. Order Items—Wigs/Cap Liners, medical I.D. Tags, etc.
   - These items I ordered when I was diagnosed. The wig was given free from the American Cancer Society through a local cancer support group. The medical I.D. states no IV's or blood pressures on surgical side (for life). The more you are able to do ahead of time, the less you forget and the less stress.

Things to Do When I'm Up

{{Place Image of calendar here, whole page}}

Things to Do When I'm Up

{{Place Image of calendar here, whole page}}

Things to Do When I'm Up

{{Place Image of calendar here, whole page}}

Housing

Bullhead City, AZ 86442 Area

Check your local listings for this information.

<u>Hud Housing:</u> (928)753-0744
809 Beale St. Ste.210
Kingman, AZ

<u>Sun River Apartments:</u> (928)763-1988
2140 Clearwater

<u>Vista Loma Apartments:</u> (928)754-5027
2367 Merrild Ave.

<u>Glenridge Apartments:</u> (928)754-4608
3475 McCormick

<u>Marble Canyon Manor:</u> (928)763-3434
1627 Mohave Dr.

<u>WACOG Appointments:</u> (928)758-3663

<u>Safe House:</u> (928)763-7233

Housing listed were ones that worked with me on my rent while trying to continue to work and going through chemo. I was able to get vouchers through a number of agencies such as: United Way, Wal-Mart, and Mohave Co. Housing Authorities.

Glossary

benign: a growth that does not leave its site of origin or invade surrounding tissue. Can get large and are capable of causing illness or even death, depending on the location of the growth.

biopsy: the examining of cells/tissues removed from a living organism. Techniques depend on the nature of the tissue and the kind of study necessary.

cancer: any malignant growth or tumor caused by abnormal and uncontrolled cell division possibly spreading to other parts of the body through the lymphatic system or the blood stream.

chemotherapy(chemo): the treatment of cancer with anticancer drugs. Drugs taken are often toxic, with severe side-effects. I also used in combination to take advantage of different modes of attack on cell division.

malignant: tumors that have the ability to invade surrounding tissues and/or spread to areas outside the local tissue. These tumors are the most dangerous and account for a large percentage of cancer deaths.

mammography: a diagnostic procedure using low-doses of X-rays to detect abnormalities in the breasts, even detecting tumors too small to be noticed on physical examination.

mastectomy: the surgical removal of breast tissue, usually done as treatment for breast cancer.

Chemo Drugs

Administered orally, in the form of an oral solution, tablets, or through injections.

Alkylating Agents: works on DNA to prevent cancer cells from reproducing, works in all phases of cell cycle.

Antimetabolites: class of drugs that interfere with DNA and RNA growth. Commonly used to treat leukemia, tumors of the breast, ovary, and the gastrointestinal tract.

Corticosteroid Hormones: steroids are natural hormones and hormone-like drugs that are useful in treating some types of cancer as well as other illnesses.

Genotoxic Agents: chemotherapy agents that affect nucleic acids and alter their function. Rapidly dividing cells are sensitive to this agent because they are actively synthesizing new DNA.

Mitotic Inhibitors: plant alkaloids and other compounds derived from natural products. Can stop mitosis or inhibit enzymes for making proteins needed for reproduction of the cell.

Nitrosoureas: interfere with enzymes that help repair DNA. These agents are able to travel from the blood to the brain.

Spindle Inhibitors: include several different chemotherapy drugs. These agents do not alter DNA structure or function, but rather the mechanics of cell division.

The following are the drugs administered while I was going through chemotherapy. Treatments were given every 21 days 4 times.

First Treatment:
Cyclophosphamide (Cytoxan., Neosar., Cytoxan., Procytox.): is an alkylating agent used singly or as a combination. Used for bladder cancer, bone cancer, cervical cancer, cancer of the adrenal cortex, endometrial cancer, lung cancer, lymphoma, prostate cancer, testicular cancer. A genotoxic agent.

Doxorubicin (Adriamycin., Rubex. and Doxil.): an anthracycline antibiotic that exerts its effects on cancer cells by intercalation and enzyme inhibition.
Colon cancer, melanoma, chronic leukemias and renal cancer show no response to this method, most others do.

Second Treatment:
Paclitaxel (Taxol., Onxol™, Paxene.): isolated compound from the Pacific Yew tree (Taxus brevifolia). Used for a variety of cancers, including ovarian, breast, small-cell and large-cell lung cancers, and Karposi's sarcoma. About 2g of paclitaxel(about 3-10 trees) treat one patient. A spindle inhibitor.

Third Treatment:
Herceptin (Trastuzumab): combined with/without paclitaxel for treatment of metastatic breast cancer whose tumors over express the HER2 (human epidermal growth factor receptor 2) protein; who have/have not received chemotherapy for their metastatic disease.

Side Effects

- Some common side effects of chemotherapy drugs include, but are not limited to:
- Acute arrhythmia
- Alopecia (hair loss)
- Amenorrhea (ending of menstrual periods)
- Birth defects (if pregnant)
- Cough
- Depression of blood cell counts
- Diarrhea
- Fever and/or chills
- Increased risk of infection and bleeding
- Irritation of the bladder
- Liver toxicity
- Loss of appetite
- Lower back or side pain
- Myelosuppression (decreased blood cell counts)
- Nausea and vomiting
- Skin and mouth ulcers
- Sterility
- Stomatitis
- Possible skin damage from previous radiation therapy
- Testicular atrophy

Patients should discuss health risks with their physician/oncologist before beginning treatments.

Websites

- **cancerquest.org**
- **getbcfacts.com (Breast Cancer)**
- **cancer.gov**
- **cancer.org**
- **webmd.com (Great for health info in general.)**
- **kidshealth.org (For parents, kids, and teens)**

Afterward

Don't mess with a menopausal woman on Chemo! It can get ugly! I was on break, eyeing a cheese cake danish in a vending machine. As it was "calling my name", I put the money in, held my breath as the spiral sprung and pushed my danish forward. Then it happened, the danish stopped, not falling. I won though, I shook the whole machine, and I got my danish. I reminded the machine—Don't mess with a menopausal woman on Chemo.

Men will experience the same. Hot flashes and night sweats are one thing but beware Chemo will magnify the ugly unfair facts. Lack of desire, depression, nausea, pain, irritability; the effects of your hormones. Happy, sad, crying, laughing, and anger.

I think there should be a singles club during Chemo. You have a better chance of finding people who understand what you're going through. I remember going through a week of identity crisis. Bald, wig, hat, bandana, which one to wear? I was very comfortable with the bald look. The pressure of a hat, wig, or other was uncomfortable.

Then the day came when I was at work and a lady customer asked me where the hair curlers were. I rubbed my bald head and said "Curlers? hum I'm not sure." She was assisted by a associate with long hair. The lady came through my register, with the curlers.

Don't adjust your vision—just like the twilight zone series. There's nothing wrong with your television, no need to adjust your screen. My vision got so blurry at times I wasn't sure what I was seeing. Had to blink a few times. Then there were the times of dry eye thank goodness for eye lubricant.

Concentration—lord, when I read about Chemo and not being able to concentrate or forgetting things the second after the fact. I was relieved to know it was not me, it was Chemo. My excuse is . . . it's Chemo just like I pleaded the fifth. My main question is, how in the world can a drug addict abuse a substance when those who want to live have to go through mild to intense treatment.

I still laugh because I refuse to let Chemo run my life. You can do it too!! Keep a positive attitude, communicate, go with the flow, and ride the wave. Surround yourself with positive people. If you run across a negative person, just give them that look and say, "Don't mess with me, I'm on Chemo!!"

Love to all of you.

what lies behind us
what lies before us
are tiny matters compared to
what lies within us

Acknowledgements

"Thank Yous"

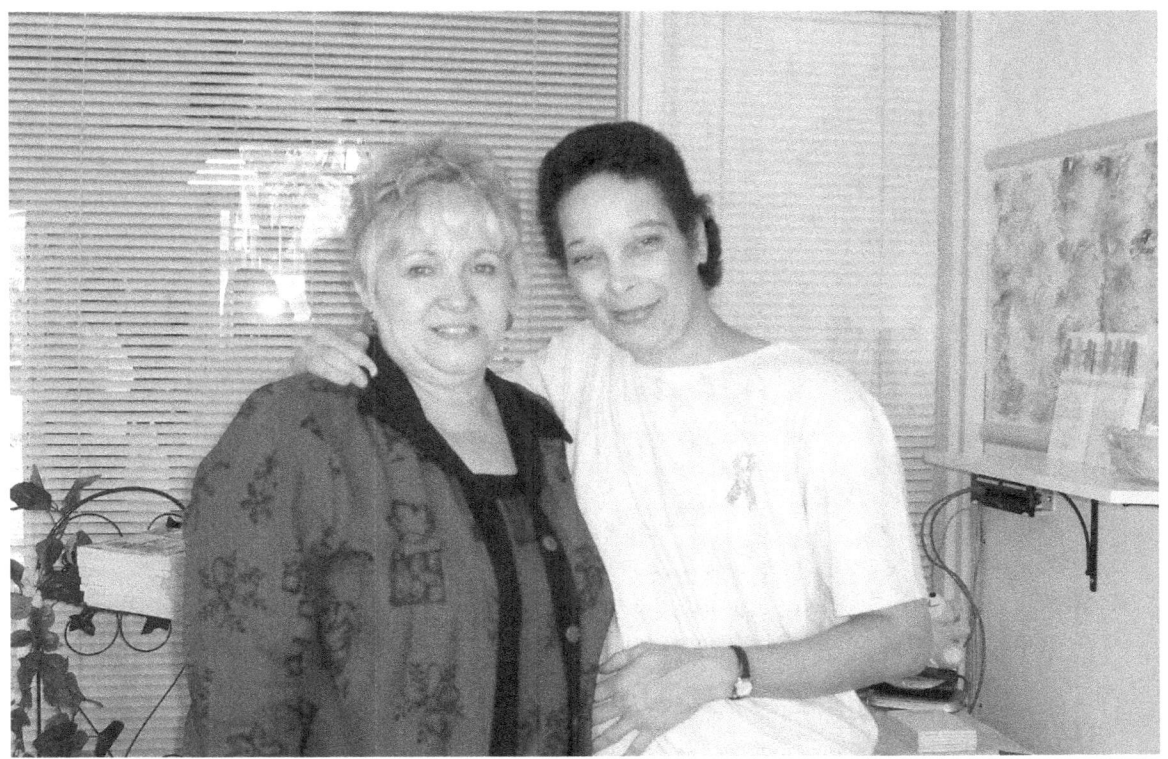

Penny Kruse for helping me in the Well Women program, being my friend.

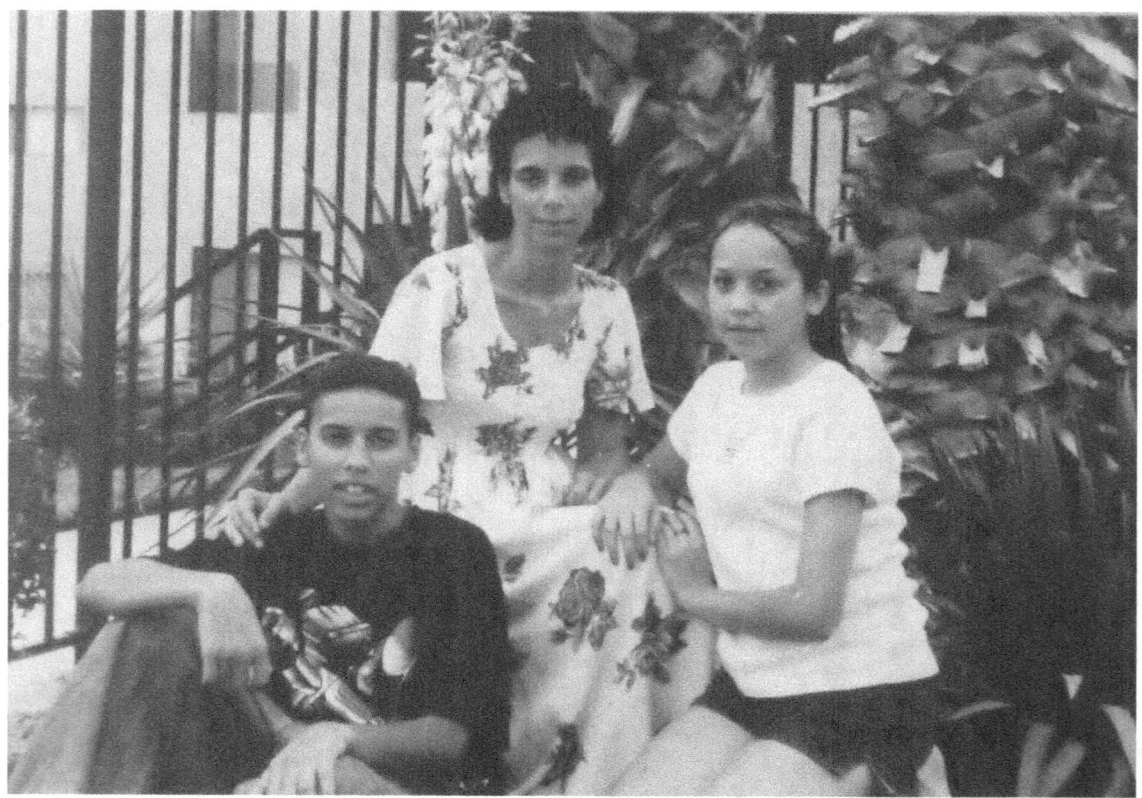

Dianne Gutierrez for listening, giving me my 1st granddaughter, helping to print this book. Christopher Gutierrez for being my son and helping me to understand life and what is really important.

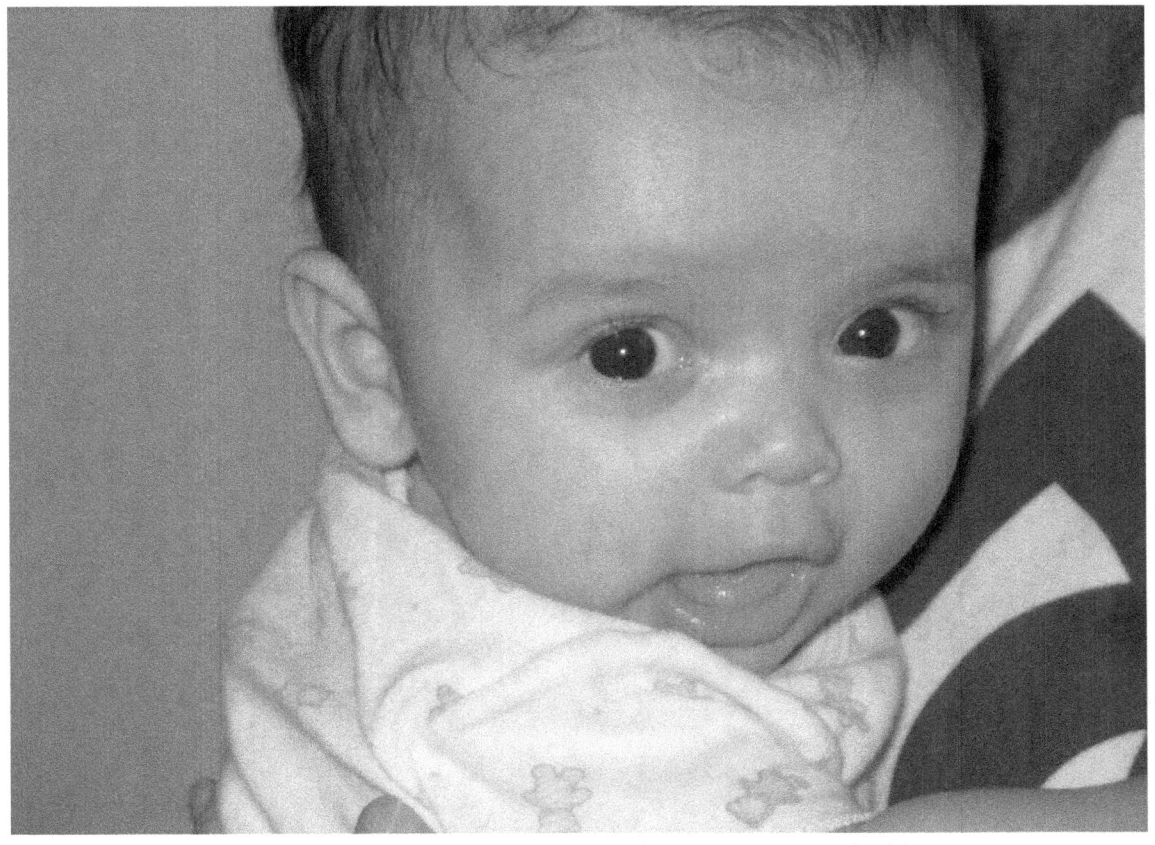

Destiny Molina for your beauty and inspiring me to hold on.

Susan-R.N. at chemo for your compassion and cheery face.

Wal-Mart #1370 for making me want to go to work.

www.ingramcontent.com/pod-product-compliance
Lightning Source LLC
Chambersburg PA
CBHW081750280526
45789CB00008B/2802